Overcome Dysthymia:

Break Free and Create a Life You Love

A Companion Guide to The Simple Success Solution

_____

NAME

_____

DATE

BOUND
PUBLISHING

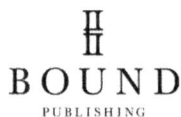

BOUND PUBLISHING

United States	Canada
6501 E. Greenway Pkwy	Suite 114
#103-480v	720 28th St. NE
Scottsdale, AZ 85254	Calgary, AB T2A 6R3

Toll Free Phone & Fax: 1-888-237-1627
Email: info@boundpublishing.com
Web: www.BoundPublishing.com
ISBN: 978-0-9867762-6-7

Library of Congress Control Number:

Cover & Text: Anamarie Seidel, Finely Finished, LLC
Edit: Lynda Masterson, Valyn Enterprises, LLC

COMPANIES, ORGANIZATIONS, INSTITUTIONS, AND INDUSTRY PUBLICATIONS. Quantity discounts are available on bulk purchases of this book for reselling, educational purposes, subscription incentives, gifts, sponsorship, or fundraising. Special books or book excerpts can also be created to fit specific needs such as private labeling with your logo on the cover and a message from a VIP printed inside. For more information, please contact our Special Sales Department at Bound Publishing.

Contents

Introduction

"What would life be if we had no courage to attempt anything?"

~ Vincent van Gogh

So let's get the obvious question out of the way—who the heck are we and why do you care? In a nutshell, we are two women who were living "normal" lives, we were successful by any societal measure and yet we were miserable—feeling stuck in our lives—*knowing* that there was more to life out there for us, but having no idea how to access it or make it happen. Then we discovered the answer. It changed *everything* in our lives.

We decided to write a book as a guide for others to achieve success in their lives, just as we had. *The Simple Success Solution* is a book that can help anyone and we are very proud of it. However, as we continued our study and began to compare our stories with those of other women, we discovered that there was a common thread that ran through the majority of them. It's that same anxious, unhappy, "stuck in a rut," knowing there's more to life story. The more we researched and studied, the more horrified we became at how prevalent depression and anxiety are in the lives of women. We *knew* that we had the solution that could help them and that it was so simple! So, we determined to develop a program that was targeted toward women like us to help them see the infinite potential within each of them and to learn to tap into it to create the life they deserve.

Take a few minutes and read our stories—they are very different, yet very similar. Do you see something of yourself in either of them? If you do we have great news—the very *best* of life is ahead of you, not behind you. You can absolutely create the life that only exists in your wildest dreams. Let us show you how!

DEB'S STORY

I have always lived what others might call a "charmed life." If I set my sights on a goal at any point in my life I achieved it, despite the odds against success. I was a straight A student, I was valedictorian of my high school class, I received my pilot's license when I was 19, I was the first female Air Force pilot to graduate from Virginia Tech, and the list goes on and on. I decided on what I wanted and then I created the favorable "breaks" needed to make it happen. I now know that I was unconsciously applying the concepts in this program all along. But what I didn't know was that my natural "goal achiever" mentality was also to be the source of a great deal of pain and frustration in my life.

When given my choice of assignments in the Air Force, I declined the more glorified roles and chose instead to become an instructor pilot. Teaching the airmen to fly T–38s was such a thrill—I could hardly believe that I was actually getting paid to do what I was doing—I loved it so much! I progressed through the ranks and ended up teaching at the U.S. Air Force Academy. It was at this point that my Air Force career started to become routine and I found myself dreaming of other things in life.

When I was 26 I married my husband, Mark—my best friend and soul mate. We were both officers in the Air Force, we were making good money, we had two beautiful daughters and were living the American Dream. I left the Air Force when my older daughter was a year old to be a full–time mother—it was my dream. In 1998, we moved back to our college town, built our dream house and Mark became a commercial airline pilot—his dream. I turned my attention to being the best mother I could be—just like my Mom had been when I was growing up. I was a volunteer parent at each of my daughter's schools, I was Brownie/Girl Scout Leader, I was a stay–at–home–mom, I baked cookies and made crafts and played Barbies. I was a *great* mom! But as time went on and my girls were in school all day, I found myself bored and stuck in a proverbial "rut." I had achieved "the American Dream"—I had it all, yet I was unfulfilled. Something was missing and to top it all off I felt like a spoiled brat, incapable of appreciating all the wonderful things in my life!

Then one day while making Christmas cookies, after 11 years of seemingly idyllic marriage, my husband broke the news that he was in love with someone else and was leaving our marriage and me. I never saw it coming and I was *crushed*. Ten days later he was gone and my world was turned completely upside down—the very act of living was an effort and I was haunted by the person I had been. I had a part–time job at a local construction company just to pass the time while the kids were at school, but suddenly, I was forced to move into a full–time position at work in order to meet my financial obligations. It wasn't long before I had completely systemized my job and there was absolutely no challenge to the work whatsoever. I was not happy, personally or professionally.

Although I had absolutely no clue at the time (and certainly would have never admitted it to myself if I had known because of the stigma I attached to it), I had slipped into a chronic, low-level depression that would last for seven years. I put up walls of security around me that only a very few people were allowed inside—I was determined that *no one* would ever hurt me again. In retrospect it is clear that my depression became a *part* of me—it was a palpable entity that affected me, my children, my friends, my job—everything. It also manifested itself in the health of my body—I was sick all the time and on numerous medications. My doctor also wrote me a prescription for an antidepressant, encouraging me to take it to just help with the anxiety and stress.

Practically everyone I knew was taking some form of antidepressant or anti–anxiety medication, so I really didn't think anything about it. I remember thinking to myself how I couldn't believe that this was my life—was this all there was to look forward to? The only thing that kept me going was my girls, who I loved above all else. I lived for those kids—spending large chunks of time volunteering at their school, flexing my work schedule around their school day and activities. They were my reason for getting out of bed each morning, but it wasn't enough. One day it struck me that perhaps I needed something for myself too. I had wanted to study karate since I was eight years old and at age 38 I finally decided to start taking classes. The study of Chinese Kempo Karate became my passion—the classes were the highlight of my days. My daughters also enrolled at the school, so it was something of a family affair. At age 42 I received my black belt. I taught most of the children's classes and ran the conditioning program for the adults. I practically lived at the karate school when I wasn't at work.

Meanwhile, I became more and more disillusioned with my job and decided to strike out on my own. I formed my own consulting company and within a couple of months was managing Virginia's only "green" building program for the western half of the state. I knew this was not my career destination, but it was a start. The next summer a friend asked me if I would participate in a free, personal development book study that he was leading. I reluctantly agreed as a favor to him. The book we studied was Napoleon Hill's *Think and Grow Rich*. I was wholly skeptical for the first few weeks, but as we delved further into the book and I began to actually study the concepts I began to wonder, "What if…" I followed that class up with a paid coaching program and my life changed forever.

As I listed the things that I really wanted in life, I realized that I was lonely, that I was tired of all the negativity—I was ready to get on with my life. I tried an experiment that was suggested—to go 30 days straight without complaining. It was amazing! With each passing week, I could feel myself changing. I was able to stop every medication that I was taking. I felt more physically and emotionally fit than I had in years—and the only thing that was different was my mindset! I was a good student, but found that the people in the coaching class were looking to me to help them through the class. The common thread through my entire life had been a sincere love and desire to teach, coach, and train people and a thought kept nagging in the back of my mind that perhaps I could combine that love with my newfound love of personal development. Over Christmas break that year, I researched the greats in personal development and was led to Bob Proctor's LifeSuccess Consultant group. After a mutual interview I signed on as a consultant and began a new direction in my life.

It was about this time when I met Angie who was the mother of one of my young karate students. We quickly became good friends and over coffee one afternoon I gave her a brief introduction to the material I taught. She immediately signed up for one of my programs and began to study under my guidance. It was such fun to watch how she latched onto these concepts and began making changes in her own life. When she left her marriage, I offered to let her and her son move in with my girls and me. We began to Mastermind on a regular basis. When I went to a consultant's training at the end of April, I was hit with a burst of intuition that Angie needed to be my partner in my business—it was only together that the company would grow and thrive. It was one of the best decisions I've ever made! Since then, we have written a book, grown our consultant business, developed a training program for other consultants, and are now focusing on helping women who are walking the same path we walked discover the life they were meant to live.

The fascinating thing that I have learned, quite recently, is that my husband leaving our marriage was not the source of my depression, although I spent plenty of time and energy blaming him for it. The heart of the matter was that I had achieved every goal I had ever set for myself throughout my life. I came to a point where I had it **all**—my dream life, or so I thought. It was the **lack** of a big huge goal in my life that was the major source of my depression—Mark was just a convenient excuse to wallow in it. I was "comfortable" in my life, but not happy, and I felt so guilty about that and the guilt just led to more unhappiness. I remember a time about a year before my marriage ended when Mark asked me what it was going to take to make me happy—what more did I want? The times I have been happiest have been when I have some "brass ring" to reach for—something to achieve, something to strive for. Starting my own business and aspiring to my first degree black belt in karate are two great examples. When I achieved a big goal I was momentarily happy—thrilled even—but over time I would have that "day after Christmas" feeling—a letdown, especially if I didn't have another goal in place to pursue.

ANGIE'S STORY

My story is about 180 degrees opposite Deb's. She was a "Stepford" child while I had something of a wild side that I explored quite extensively, much to my parents' chagrin. She became the first female Air Force pilot from our alma mater—I changed majors twice and dropped out after three years. She made her own breaks, I went with the flow and the status quo was my friend—or so I thought. She achieved whatever goal she set out to—I never quite felt that I measured up. You see, I was born when my parents were 18 years old. My Dad was like Deb—he knew what he wanted and he found a way to make it happen. He was a perfect student, was accepted into Harvard Law School when he was 30 years old, had a brilliant career in banking law and retired at age 55 to do whatever the heck he wanted to do. My Mom stayed home with my sister and me and put all her dreams on hold to help my Dad make his come true. In my first 12 years, my family was constantly financially strapped—money was always an issue. My self–image formed with a whole collection of baggage and bad habits around money, and relationships, and self worth and what I believed I was capable of doing. I was always compared to my father—the way I looked, the way I thought, the way I approached things, but I never measured up to him—at least not in my own mind.

I did do some things that I am proud of though. After leaving college at 20 years of age, I moved to New York City and lived there quite successfully for four years. I figured if I could "make it there, I could make it anywhere"—and I did, and it was a blast! I left New York for a consulting job that sent me to Southern California for six months and then to Davenport, Iowa for a year. I didn't like living in the Midwest at all and I was completely *alone* for the first time in my life. My fiancé was a Corpsman in the Navy stationed on an aircraft carrier in the middle of the Persian Gulf during the first Gulf War, so it wasn't like he was available for phone calls very often, and email and instant messaging were still several years away. I decided to move back to my hometown and finish college and went on to earn a Master's degree as well. My fiancé, Mark, soon after became my husband and life was good. However, it became apparent after several months that Mark had a drinking problem and a responsibility issue, but I loved him and figured if I loved him enough he would change.

When we had been married about seven years, we decided it was time to start a family. Unfortunately, it wasn't as easy as they tell you when you're a teenager! It took three and a half years of concerted effort, tests, surgeries, and "scheduling" (if you know what I mean) before I found out on December 21, 2001 that I was pregnant. That was a great time in my life. Joshua was born exactly one week late on September 9, 2002 after a 24-hour labor. He has been my greatest achievement in life, no doubt about it. I was in a pretty happy place—I had the baby I wanted, a husband who was intent on being a good dad, a home, two cars, good jobs—by all measure we were successful. Infertility takes a toll on a marriage though. There is no better way to strip every bit of passion out of a marriage than to plan your sex life around a calendar or the color on a stick for years on end! Mark and I started on a slow downward spiral not long after Josh was born. Not that there weren't good times—there were—*many* of them, but Mark's drinking got worse, he stayed out later and later. We bought a new home when Josh was a year old and went into a huge amount of debt outfitting the house with everything we "needed." I kept trying to piece together a solution to our financial problems, but when more is going out each month than is coming in, it's not a good situation.

I found myself in a place where I had no social life, no outside activities; my son was my life and my life revolved around his schedule. I suffered from low self-esteem, anxiety, fatigue and just felt lost and useless much of the time. Because I had a husband who was more and more absent, I was lonely and miserable—and I felt *guilty* as hell for feeling miserable, because I was so much better off than most of the people I knew! But in the final analysis I felt like I was sprinting on a treadmill every single day, with life passing me by, but being unable to keep up with it.

In 2006 Mark had a *bad* car accident—he had an incredible amount of alcohol in his system. Luckily, no one else was involved, but his truck was unrecognizable and he is quite lucky that he wasn't killed. He was cut up and bruised and had some nerve damage, but physically there was no permanent damage. He was, however, charged with driving while intoxicated and there were numerous fines and he lost his driver's license for a year. He promised me that his drinking days were over and I had hopes that this was his "bottom" and that change would really happen. Unfortunately, it didn't work out that way. Once the physical injuries had healed he was back in the bars and I admittedly enabled his behavior by providing transportation. I told him that I would walk through hell with him once, but if he was ever caught drinking and driving again, I would leave him—I wouldn't put myself or our son through it again.

Over the next couple of years I became increasingly unhappy. I kept talking to myself saying that I had to figure out a way to be okay with my life because this is just what it *was* for the foreseeable future. The debt kept mounting and Mark kept his social calendar full and I was alone with my son most of the time. I found myself turning to alcohol to just take the edge off at the end of the day—before long, more evenings than not I found myself at the bottom of a bottle of wine. I was highly functional—I never missed work or slacked off at home or ignored my son or my responsibilities, but I was in a very bad place. I was gaining weight at a rapid rate, I was miserable and I was laser focused on all the problems in my life—no wonder I was broke, unhealthy and unhappy!

I have to say that I put on a very good face for the rest of the world though. No one, not even my closest family and friends, knew the depth of my problems. I was scared and I ached to just feel "normal!" I met Deb in January at the karate school where Josh took classes. She approached me one day in January and that conversation changed the course of my life.

We talked for a long time while Josh was taking a class and she told me her story. I felt a connection to her and I wanted to know more, so I asked her out for coffee and she shared some information with me that transformed my way of thinking. See, she showed me in 20 minutes how my thoughts—my focus on my problems—were actually creating more of the same problems. My focus was on lack, loss and limitation instead of abundance, increase and possibility. There was an audible "click" in my head as she spoke and I knew I had found the answers I was so desperately searching for. She became my personal development coach that day and I have not looked back!

In March, my husband was arrested for a second driving under the influence charge and I found the strength and courage to leave my marriage of almost 18 years. I made a decision to get healthy and lost 30 pounds and started an exercise program (including studying karate myself) and am in better physical condition than I have ever been in. I made the decision to stop drinking for comfort, and now will only drink on occasion to enjoy the flavor. I made the decision to get my finances in order and paid off a mountain of debt. I joined forces with Deb as a partner in her personal development consulting business and we both quit our passionless "jobs" and now spend our days doing what we love to do. I am a better mother, partner, friend and person now that I am living the life I was destined for—it is fuller and richer than I ever imagined possible.

It has taken me 45 years to get me to the point where I can honestly say that I love who I am—I love *me*! It's no wonder I have left a trail of bad relationships in my wake over my lifetime. You can't give what you don't have. You can't love someone if you don't love yourself first.

What a difference a year can make! We are writing this workbook around the holidays and it seems to be a time for personal reflection. I've been looking back on my progress over the past year and thought it worth sharing. *There is **nothing** exceptional about my progress or achievements this year. I just latched onto the principles that Deb and I now teach and applied them to my life and things began to happen with such speed and regularity that it was frightening sometimes. This type of change can happen for you too!*

MY FINANCIAL LIFE

Last Christmas I found myself in a terrible predicament financially—my husband and I were in more debt than we could seemingly *ever* possibly pay back. We had two mortgages and five credit cards between us (which were soon to be maxed out because there was a small child to buy presents for who would not understand why the recession hit Santa so hard.) Our monthly outflow was exceeding our inflow. We were in a bad place and I was scared to death. My thoughts focused on *how* I could get out of debt. Our financial crisis was at the center of my thoughts.

This Christmas, I am debt–free, my home is for sale, Christmas presents were purchased with cash and are wrapped and either under the tree or ready for Santa to deliver on Christmas morning. I can't believe the complete 180-degree turnaround that has occurred! My thoughts are focused on abundance and the possibilities for the future.

MY RELATIONSHIP

Last Christmas my marriage was falling apart. I was as emotionally bankrupt as I was financially. My husband was drinking heavily and staying out very late—often not even coming home until I was getting ready to leave for work in the morning. One particular morning I recall him coming home in a really nasty mood—it was very unpleasant. As I drove my son to school that morning and myself to my "job" I vividly remember marveling to myself "is this *really* my life?" I had such high ambitions for what I wanted to be, do and have and look what my life had become!

This Christmas I am nine months into the separation of my marriage. I have a new relationship, which is more wonderful than anything I could have possibly dreamed. I feel supported and loved for who I am at my core. I am valued just for being me. I feel whole and free, maybe for the first time in my entire adult life.

MY CAREER

Last Christmas I was two months into my 13th year in my job as a program manager at a state university and I felt fortunate to have such a "safe" position. However, I no longer enjoyed my job. It was harder and harder to jump out of bed in the morning, excited about the day ahead. In fact, more often than not I truly *dreaded* it. Plus, I was grossly underpaid. It was a depressing prospect that this was my lot in life for the next 17 years!

This Christmas I own my own business. I am a published author. I am writing a second book right now. I am developing personal growth programs that will impact women's lives all over the world. I collaborate with people around the globe every day. I *do* jump out of bed excited for what the day has in store for me. I left my "job" behind in August and have found my passion and my purpose in my career today. I love it so much!

MY HEALTH AND WELLBEING

Last Christmas I would end about five out of every seven days at the bottom of a bottle of wine. I was drinking so much that I honestly hardly even felt it after drinking a whole bottle of wine and that really scared me. At 5'5" tall, I weighed 175 lbs. and was gaining weight every month. I was completely inactive—the most exercise I got was walking to the mailbox each day. I sat in the karate school where my son took classes and made excuses for why I couldn't take classes as well. I was miserable, depressed and felt like the best of life was well behind me. My son was the only thing that gave me joy.

This Christmas I weigh 145 pounds, I work out hard four to five days per week. I decided to join the karate school last January and fell in love with the study of martial arts immediately. I am currently working toward my green belt and am considered one of the most physically fit students in the school—even at the age of 45! I did not eliminate wine from my life, but I have moderated drastically. Deb and I will share a nice bottle of wine on Saturdays as a treat. It's a special time just for us, but I have no need to numb my feelings any longer. I know beyond a shadow of a doubt that the best of life lies ahead of me!

As you can see we are no different than any of you reading this book. We have experienced times of incredible highs and devastating lows, we have had great success and dismal failures, we have been ruled by our emotions and succumbed to crippling negativity. What sets us apart is that both of us reached a point in our lives where we stopped and told ourselves that enough was enough. We knew that there was more to life than what we were living. We knew that if we were open to a solution it would present itself—and it *did*!

Developing an understanding of the laws that dictate the way the world works—laws as steadfast and unchangeable as the Law of Gravity—allowed us to see that everything that was affecting and shaping our lives—people, circumstances, possessions, opportunities, etc. were all of our own making. They were our responsibility as surely as if we were the potter at the wheel, sculpting the physical manifestations in our lives with our very hands.

So, don't beat yourself up if your life is not what you would like it to be. It's okay and it's not your fault! The concepts you will learn in this book are not new—they are thousands of years old—it is just that most people have never been introduced to them before. We have taken the best from the world of personal development and distilled it into a system that will empower you to create the life of your dreams!

So, sit back, read, learn and awaken the creative muse that is crying out within you right now. You'll be amazed at what will happen.

Sincerely,

DEB CHESLOW   ANGIE FLYNN

Normal Is HIGHLY Overrated!

"Normal is not something to aspire to, it's something to get away from."
—Jodie Foster

So what is normal anyway? The dictionary defines it as:

Normal

1. Conforming to the standard or the common type; usual; not abnormal; regular; natural.

2. Serving to establish a standard.

Society says that normal is that state of being where we are happy and carefree, we have great jobs that pay well, we have happy relationships or growing families, we have the great house we always wanted and the cars we dreamed of since we were kids. But, if this is true then it would appear that there is a new standard of "normal" coming into existence, and it is one of chronic depression.

THE STATISTICS

According to a Harvard Medical Center study, the rate of depression is doubling every 20 years, with a current rate of approximately 18.8 million American adults, or about nine and a half per cent of the U.S. population age 18 and older, being affected by depressive disorders in a given year.

According to the National Institute of Mental Health, approximately 12.4 million women in the U.S. each year suffer from a depressive disorder; it seems like a lot of women are all in the same boat! By the standard mentioned above we're doing well—decent jobs, nice houses and such but yet we feel guilty as hell and we're miserable! In a National Mental Health Association survey, 41% of depressed women reported that they were too embarrassed to seek help. In an effort to abate the misery, some are turning to a couple of drinks at the end of the day; while others are popping antidepressants to take the edge off. According to the Center for Disease Control, adult use of antidepressants had almost tripled between 1994 and 2000 with over ten percent of women 18 and older now taking antidepressants. It seems like just about every woman we know is taking some form of antidepressant or anti–anxiety medication—Deb was one of them!

"In 2002, more than one in three doctor's office visits by women involved a prescription for an antidepressant," says Amy Bernstein, Center for Mental Health Services of the Centers for Disease Control and Prevention. A full 70% of the prescriptions written for antidepressant medications are written for women. Can you imagine? Women are going to the doctor for a headache and walking out with a script for an antidepressant! It's ridiculous!

DYSTHYMIA: MYTH OR MONSTER?

Chronic, low–level depression has reached such epidemic proportions that the medical community has given it a name—Dysthymia (pronounced dis-*thigh*-me-ah). It's a big problem affecting nearly 8% of the U.S. population. Low-grade depression (dysthymia) is one of the most common ailments on the planet and one of the least likely to be diagnosed. Like its cousin, clinical depression, low–grade depression hits women roughly twice as often as men. Dysthymia is, by definition, chronic. A diagnosis requires the presence of symptoms on more days than not for a period of at least two years, which is what makes it so hard to pin down. Any given day might be okay, even happy. Yet in the general run of days, there are more gray ones than not, more unhappiness than joy. Most people afflicted with this kind of chronic malaise instinctively blame themselves: They would rather believe they can solve the problem—if they could just find the right job or the right man or lose weight—than admit they have a psychiatric disorder. Unfortunately, many people who are suffering do not seek help because they have been feeling this way for so long, the feelings of depression and malaise are their "normal".

The presence of two or more of the following symptoms persisting for at least two years is indicative of dysthymia in adults:

- Poor appetite or overeating

- Insomnia or hypersomnia

- Low energy or fatigue

- Low self–esteem

- Poor concentration

- Difficulty making decisions

- Feelings of hopelessness

DEPRESSION SELF–ASSESSMENT

Read the following statements. Think about the past two weeks and check the statements that describe you during this timeframe?

- ❑ My sleep patterns are all messed up (i.e. having trouble falling asleep, waking up constantly through the night, or oversleeping in the morning).

- ❑ I feel uninterested in the things that were once enjoyable to me.

- ❑ I just feel sad.

- ❑ I tend to ignore the phone when it rings even though it may be one of my friends.

- ❑ I have no energy.

- ❑ I've been crying a lot.

- ❑ It seems like everything goes wrong no matter how hard I try.

- ❑ I turn down social invitations because I feel I have nothing to offer the group and that my bad mood would just bring everyone else down.

- ❑ I purposely engage in risky behavior such as crossing the street against the light.

- ❑ I skip work or school because I feel depressed.

- ❑ I just can't seem to make a decision.

- ❑ I feel like a failure and that I'm letting my friends and family down.

- ❑ I hurt! I have a constant headache or stomachache or my joints hurt, even though there is no apparent cause.

- ❑ I think about death a lot.

- ❑ I've gained or lost weight without really trying.

- ❑ I can't concentrate for any length of time.

- ❑ I have thought about purposely hurting myself.

- ❑ I've been drinking more alcohol than usual.

- ❑ I have no interest in sex or am experiencing sexual difficulties.

- ❑ I have a very short fuse—I get irritated easily.

- ❑ Eating seems to be more trouble than it's worth.

How many boxes did you check? If it's more than five then you are not living the life you were destined for. Creating a life beyond your wildest imaginations does not have to be a struggle or a burden! It's simple and we can show you how to be, do, and have more in your life.

So, what's the problem? Why are so many women having such an issue with anxiety and/or depression? One reasons is that we are taught and conditioned from our first day on this planet to go after "the American Dream" (or the European dream, or the Australian Dream—or whatever—you get our point)— to have it *all*—the family, the relationship, the career, the house, car, money, etc. Over time, one of two things seems to happen—either you fall short in one or more areas of life and eventually give up on your dreams (like Angie), or you actually ***get*** it all and find yourself in this place of comfort and routine with no new goals on the horizon (like Deb). In either case, you find yourself in a dark place where you feel absolutely stuck and dissatisfied with your life and if left unchecked, that dissatisfaction has a nasty way of manifesting itself as chronic, low level depression.

The mental health experts have identified all kinds of underlying factors why women, in particular, are so susceptible to developing depression in their middle years. According to the National Institute of Mental Health, women develop depression at more than twice the rate of men. We've boiled these factors down into six basic areas:

1. *Frazzlemania* (**Overload**): The demands on women today are ***huge***! Most middle-aged women have careers, families, households, aging parents and a myriad of other responsibilities vying for their time and attention. Striking a balance between all of them has a tendency to leave one feeling like a failure—spend too much time on the career and the children suffer— too much time on the kids and the marriage suffers—you can see the problem. Plus, many women were born at a time when it was very common for women to be stay–at–home–moms and there is guilt in play as well when they feel they are not doing as good a job managing everything as their own mother did. The guilt, coupled with the sense of failure and stress, make a fertile ground for depression to take root.

2. *2nd Class Setback* (**Societal Gender Inequity**): As evolved as we would like to think we are, the fact remains that in much of the industrialized world, women are often still not valued at the same level as men. Women who do not work outside the home are often perceived as sitting around watching soap operas and eating bonbons during the day. Women who do take time away from their careers to raise children have a difficult, if not impossible, time making up lost ground in terms of pay and retirement savings. These types of "no–win" scenarios can lead women to feel like second-class citizens and cause stress and hopelessness.

3. ***Foggy Glasses Syndrome:*** Depression is very much a disease of perception. Everywhere we look are images of perfection—the perfect body, the perfect car, the perfect house, the perfect relationship, the perfect children, etc. Perfection is an illusion, yet everyone is trying to attain it. These images are hard to live up to at any age, but become particularly glaring as we age. Constant exposure to these images of perfection works on us in subtle, subconscious ways making us feel "less than".

4. ***The Sucker Punch*** (Traumatic Life Events): How we react to unexpected events in life certainly affects our mood and emotions. A stressful life event can plunge a person into depression, especially if a person is at risk for depression due to other factors. Stressful life events may include: prolonged medical illness; illness or death of a loved one; divorce; ending a close relationship; loss of a job; relocating; and financial or legal problems.

5. ***The Clone-Effect*** (Environmental Factors): The environment in which you were raised can be a major factor underlying your susceptibility to depression. If you were raised to think you were never good enough or that you were a "bad" kid or other negative ideas, these ideas are incorporated into your self-image over time. If you have a negative self-image, the twists and turns of life can make you much more susceptible to becoming depressed.

6. ***Comfortitis*** (Comfort vs. Achievement): Think back to Deb's story. She was a goal achiever from Day One—she always wanted to be doing it better, faster, smarter than anyone thought possible. Once she got to a point in her life where she had achieved the major goals she had set for herself, she became "comfortable" and in that "comfort", found herself utterly miserable. People like Deb need to constantly be striving for the next goal—without it, they feel rudderless, without purpose, and depression can easily take hold.

Regardless of the underlying factor (or factors) that caused it, the first step in getting through the depression is to admit that there is a problem. Seriously, isn't it sad that so many women just can't wait to get together with their friends on the weekends to compare complaints? We know we relished those "bull sessions!" How many conversations did we have with ourselves saying that we had to find a way to be okay with our lives, to accept it—this was just the way it was! Well, pardon our bluntness, but that's a load of crap! The life you are living right now is ***not*** the way it ***has*** to be! You are not a slave to your circumstances!

Sadly, everyone will at some time in their life be affected by depression, whether it be their own or someone else's. Fifty-four percent of those people believe depression is a personal weakness and that there is no hope for them to get through it, which is why 80% of people suffering from chronic, low level depression are not currently having any treatment. And get this, A National Mental Health Association survey showed that more than 50% of women believe depression is a "normal part of aging" and that treatment for depression during menopause is not necessary!

According to the World Health Organization depression is the second largest killer of man, after heart disease, with studies showing that depression is a contributory factor to fatal coronary disease. *and* current projections show depression overtaking heart disease as the #1 killer worldwide by the year 2020. There have even been studies done showing links between depression and illness including osteoporosis, diabetes, heart disease, some forms of cancer, eye disease and back pain.

But you know, we just don't pay as much attention to our mental health and well-being as we do our physical health. We read those statistics and most of us just shrug and say there is nothing I can do about it, that's just life. Well, in part, that's true. It *is* your life and that is because everything we do, every feeling we have and our belief system and the programming we received as a child are driving every result we are getting. That self-image, that belief system, is nothing more than a huge collection of habits—the programming. It's happening in the background and without your permission. It's like a computer virus. Those little bugs get inside your computer and wreak havoc, but they don't keep you from using your computer until things get so bad that the system just crashes. They operate in the background, not caring what you try to do, they just carry out their program unbeknownst to you. So how do you keep from becoming a statistic? Is there a way to change your programming?

The cool thing is that it really *is* possible and actually quite simple to re-program your "hard drive" with clean, virus-free programs of your choosing! We remember feeling angry when we learned how simple it all is and that we hadn't been taught this information before. There's nothing new about it—no big stroke of brilliance on our part—it's been around for thousands of years, but it's stuff that isn't taught in school—although it certainly should be!

That feeling that life is hopeless or out of control, being angry at yourself for not being able to do anything about it, changes in sleep or eating habits, loss of interest in engaging in activities that once gave you joy—we've convinced ourselves that all of these are normal parts of life. We convince ourselves further that as long as we are not under a doctor's care or on prescription medications that everything is okay. But the fact is that these are all signs that something is wrong and the cause can be traced back to some "virus" in your mind. The emotional pain that you feel is the higher side of yourself screaming at you to live up to your infinite potential—to do more, be more, have more!

There is help out there! Traditional programs for stress and behavior modification get you all hyped up with motivation, but offer no follow through action plan. Think of the typical diet program—it teaches you how to modify your behavior to eat in a certain way, to exercise a certain way, but fails to address the root cause of the excess weight—the self-image—the ***programming!*** For lasting change to occur the cause of the problem has to be tackled, not just the symptoms.

It is your birthright to be happy and prosperous and your obligation to be all you can possibly be. Why on earth should we settle for the status quo when greatness and abundance beyond our wildest dreams is within our grasp? Complete the exercises below and read on to find out how you can empower yourself to a better life!

MEET ALLY

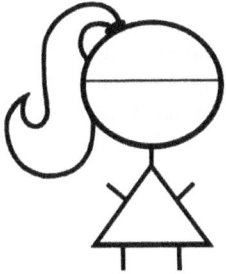

Ally is a 40-year-old woman who has been married to the same man for nearly 20 years. She works for a large law firm in a paralegal position that she doesn't particularly enjoy, but she has seniority and it pays pretty well. She dreamed of going to law school when she was younger, but chose to put those dreams on hold when she met Jack. They married and quickly had Emily and William, who are now teenagers. She and Jack own their home in the suburbs, own nice cars and have built a small nest egg in the bank. Ally has many friends and some outside activities that keep her busy. Over the past several years, however, Ally has been plagued by this empty feeling. She thinks about her family and feels so guilty that she keeps wondering if the best of her life is behind her. She thinks about her long abandoned hopes and aspirations for her life wistfully and wonders if there isn't more for her out there somewhere. She gets together with her girlfriends and they all sit around and rehash the negative things that are happening in their lives. When she leaves these get-togethers she feels even worse. She hasn't been sleeping well for months, hasn't been eating right and finds herself having a few glasses of wine in the evening just to take the day's edge off. She feels exhausted, anxious, sad, lonely and worst of all, guilty for her feelings.

As we proceed through the workbook, we'll periodically check in with Ally as an example, working through the exercises.

EXERCISE 1: THE "LOOK IN THE MIRROR" QUIZ

The first, and often hardest, step in the process is admitting that there is a problem. How do you determine whether or not dysthymia is affecting your life? Here are a few simple questions to help determine if this program is for you.

How has each of the following issues affected you?

1. Little interest or pleasure in doing things.

_____

_____

2. Feeling down, depressed or hopeless.

_____

_____

3. Longing for more or wondering if the best of life is behind you.

_____

_____

4. Trouble falling/staying asleep or sleeping too much.

_____

_____

5. Feeling tired or having little energy.

_____

_____

6. Feeling stressed, anxious, or frazzled by the end of the day.

_____

_____

7. Feeling overwhelmed.

_____

_____

8.   Feeling inadequate or like a "second-class" citizen.

_____

_____

9.   Poor appetite or overeating.

_____

_____

10.   Feeling bad about yourself, that you are a failure or have let yourself or your family down.

_____

_____

11.   Trouble concentrating on things, such as reading the newspaper or watching television.

_____

_____

12.   Moving or speaking very slowly or being fidgety or restless, trying to feel purposeful.

_____

_____

13.   Feeling that you need to have a drink or take medication to make the feelings go away.

_____

_____

There are two things you need to get clear on if you want to change your life: where you are and where you want to go. The purpose of the previous exercise is not to make you dwell on your problems, but to gain some clarity on where you are right now. In the next chapter we will start looking at where you want to go. You know, sometimes we can be our own worst enemy– we tend to let our circumstances and our very state of mind place artificial limitations on our lives. Next, let's spend a little bit of time thinking about those circumstantial limitations.

EXERCISE 2: CIRCUMSTANTIAL OR SELF–IMPOSED LIMITATIONS

If you truly *want* more out of life then ponder the next few questions to get you thinking about the limitations you may be placing on yourself and how those feelings of limitation are being expressed (through actions or in the health of your physical body),

1.   Do you feel "stuck" in your career or are you working in a job that is frustrating or dissatisfying simply because you don't believe you could find something more fulfilling or because you have too much time vested in the position or the company?

_____

_____

2.   Ask the same question about your relationships.

_____

_____

3.   Are you not fully opening yourself up in your relationships (especially partnerships, marriages, etc.) for fear of getting hurt or being rejected?

_____

_____

4.   Have you given up on a dream, such as one of furthering your education, because of the "realities" that there is no time or money for such luxuries?

_____

_____

5.   Do you fear failure? Does this fear prevent you from stepping out and testing new ground, trying new things, learning new things?

_____

_____

6.   How do you perceive yourself? What are your greatest strengths? Your most limiting weaknesses?

_____

_____

7.   What are you afraid of? What thoughts keep you awake at night?

_____

_____

8.   What are some dreams for your life that you had when you were young which you have abandoned on over the years? If it were impossible to fail, would you still want to realize those dreams?

_____

_____

9.   Describe yourself using 10 adjectives or roles.

_____

_____

10.   List 10 adjectives or roles you would *like* to be described by.

_____

_____

11.   Are you overly concerned with what other people think of you or how they perceive you (guess what—it's none of your business what other people think of you!)?

_____

_____

12.   How do you talk to yourself? What are the conversations that go on in your head? Do you tell yourself how smart and worthy and wonderful you are or do you focus on more negative things ("Oh, another diet? Don't you know you're doomed to fail—*again?*"... "Don't even bother applying for that job—you couldn't possibly do it—you're not good enough?"... "Karate? You? Are you nuts?") (*Yeah, I know a little something about negative inner dialogue! –A*)

_____

_____

_____

_____

We'll get into the nuts and bolts of all this in the following chapters, but for right now just know that these things you've identified as self-limiting behaviors or habits are really **_not_** your fault! They are the result of your self-image—a whole collection of beliefs and habits that make you who you are. Your self-image was formed a long time ago with very little or no input from you, which kind of stinks if you have a not so great self-image! In his program "Lead the Field," Earl Nightingale said something quite profound: "Now, right here we come to a rather interesting fact, we tend to minimize the things we can do, the goals we can reach, and for some equally strange reason we think other people can accomplish things we cannot." He's talking about the kind of limiting cross talk that you have with yourself every single day! The fantastic news is that you can re-program your self-image to be whatever you want it to be. Stick with us and we'll show you how!

It is important that you realize that you only get **_one life_**! This is not a dress rehearsal, you only get "one bite at the apple" (as our dear friend Bob Proctor is so fond of saying)—your life should be big and beautiful and **_everything_** you want it to be! Think about how you spend your days… each and every day you are literally trading your life for what you do, the people you associate with, the job you go to. Is the life you have currently worth **_dying_** for? If it's not, don't feel bad—most people are in the very same boat. Keep reading, pour your heart and soul into the exercises in this book and let us show you how to break free from the bonds of dysthymia, embrace change and create a life you truly love!

Turn Your Dreamers On

"We are what we think.
All that we are arises with our thoughts.
With our thoughts, we make the world."
~ Buddha

Before we go on, take a moment and answer a few questions.

1.   Think back to when you were a child, what did you want to be when you grew up?

_____

_____

_____

2.   What did you dream of achieving when you were in high school or college?

_____

_____

_____

3.   What dreams have you given up on over the years as you "grew up" and got realistic?

_____

_____

_____

Have you ever noticed how great children are at using their imagination and dreaming? You give them a cabinet full of Tupperware or pots and pans and they can turn those pieces into musical instruments, spaceships, buildings, blocks—you name it. Children have a natural ability to tap into one of their most powerful intellectual faculties, which is their imagination. Unfortunately, along about five to six years of age, that same child—let's call her Jill—is sent off to school and while sitting in her classroom listening to her teacher go on and on about something she needs to "know," she looks out the window and starts daydreaming about a game of hop-scotch or something and all of a sudden—wham!! The teacher's hand slams down on her desk and she is told to "Stop daydreaming! Pay attention! You're not a baby anymore— it's time to grow up!" Slowly but surely, over the coming 10–15 years, the "dreamers" in that child are shut down and Jill becomes logical and realistic and reasonable. She lets go of all the big, beautiful "what if" dreams she had for her life and chooses a safe, predictable path. Jill lives her life quite successfully—she has a husband, a couple of children, a nice house in the suburbs, a couple of nice cars in the garage, plenty of money in the bank, a membership at the Country Club—by all societal measures she is living the American Dream! So, why does Jill find herself sobbing in the shower with a bottle of antidepressants in the medicine chest and an empty bottle of wine in the kitchen more nights than not. Why is Jill miserable in her seemingly perfect life?

When we stop dreaming or let go of the dreams we have of what we want our life to be, we lose connection with our spiritual side—our higher self—that sense of oneness with infinite power. This can cause us great psychological pain and anxiety. Plus there is a part of our subconscious that is actually pissed off at us for giving up on our dreams. This anger is turned inward and can manifest itself in all sorts of nasty ways, including anxiety and depressive disorders. So, how do we reconnect with our higher self? It's simple (although not necessarily easy)! We have to start dreaming and creating and using our imagination again! We know when we heard this we thought, "Well, duh! But how do we do that?" You see, when you get to middle age and are so used to not dreaming and imagining, it can be difficult to crank up those creaky, rusty dream machines in our minds. But believe us, it is so worth it!

One area scientists have been making advances in is the area of thought process. According to a 2009 issue of Psychology Today, brain studies now reveal that thoughts produce the same mental instructions as physical actions. Mental imagery impacts many cognitive processes in the brain: motor control, attention, perception, planning, and memory. So the brain is getting trained for actual performance during visualization. It's been found that mental practices can enhance motivation, increase confidence and self-efficiency, improve motor performance, prime your brain for success, and increase states of flow—all relevant to achieving your best life!

Genevieve Behrend, author of *Your Invisible Power* has much to say on this topic. She writes, "The exercise of the visualizing faculty keeps your mind in order, and attracts to you the things you need to make life more enjoyable in an orderly way. If you train yourself in the practice of deliberately picturing your desire and carefully examining your picture, you will soon find that your thoughts and desires proceed in a more orderly procession than ever before. Having reached a state of ordered mentality, you are no longer in a constant state of mental hurry. Hurry is Fear, and consequently destructive. In other words, when your understanding grasps the power to visualize your heart's desire and hold it with your will, it attracts to you all things requisite to the fulfillment of that picture by the harmonious vibrations of the Law of Attraction. You realize that since Order is Heaven's first law, and visualization places things in their natural order, then it must be a heavenly thing to visualize. Everyone visualizes, whether he knows it or not. Visualizing is the great secret of success. The conscious use of this great power attracts to you multiplied resources, intensifies your wisdom, and enables you to make use of advantages which you formerly failed to recognize."

Isn't that beautiful? What she is saying, in a nutshell, is that visualizing allows you to tap into the spiritual side of your nature, ordering your thoughts and allowing you to be calm. When you are in touch with your oneness with Infinite Power (whatever that means to you—God, science, energy, etc.) you are able to attract that which you require to make your vision a reality.

The Law of Vibration and its sub–law, the Law of Attraction are so powerful! At its most basic level this law states that everything at its most basic is energy and energy vibrates on a frequency. Thoughts are energy as well and they also vibrate on a frequency and like energy attracts like energy. The Law of Attraction states that "like attracts like."

For the purposes of creating the life you want to live, it is important that you grasp one very basic truth: Your current life, your current circumstances are a manifestation of your past thoughts and feelings. This is what is so awesome! You can decide, right here and right now to change your life by changing what you are consistently thinking about. If you "think" about it (no pun intended), what do most people dwell on in their mind? What they want in life or what they don't want in life? When you are lying awake in the middle of the night, what are the thoughts that are creeping through your mind—what are the pictures you are painting with those thoughts? For Angie, it was very much thoughts about her broken marriage and her lack of financial resources and how she was doomed to this life of misery. For Deb, it was thoughts of hurt and betrayal by someone she dearly loved. You see, we use our thoughts in a backwards manner—we're constantly focusing on what we don't want and then we're shocked when we get more and more of it!

The Law of Attraction responds to the emotions behind the thoughts. Those emotions could be good or bad; the Law doesn't care. If you really want something and feel really good about it, you will most likely get it. On the other hand, if you do not want something at all, and feel bad about the prospect of having it, you will probably get it, too! The Law of Attraction is all-inclusive. Whatever is most prominent in your awareness is the actual thing you are going to attract. The way that this happens is through focused thought and through feeling.

Your feelings will tell you what you are attracting. If you aren't sure how you're feeling, just take a look at your present results. If you are thinking and feeling good, you will be attracting good stuff. If you are thinking and feeling bad, you will be attracting bad stuff; it is as simple as that.

So, we want to visualize the things we really want and then feel what it feels like to actually have what we're visualizing. There are lots of ways to help this process along, but first, you have to actually decide what you really want.

The next exercise will take you through this process, but let us be very clear here—we're not talking about what you think you can get—we're talking heart's desire stuff here. After you've determined what you want, you have to start thinking about it and really getting emotionally involved with the idea of actually having it. You have to start thinking about it as having already manifested in your life. Now, this may get uncomfortable and we'll go into why in the next chapter, but it is essential that you attach as much positive emotion as you possibly can to your want.

One thing we have done is to actually record our vision statement on a digital recorder. We play those recordings first thing every morning and the last thing every night. The statement is read in the present tense—as if the goal has already been attained. We talk about how it feels to have what we want and what a day in this new life is like—in as much detail as we can muster.

There is something very powerful that happens subconsciously when you listen to your vision read in your own voice as having already manifested!

EXERCISE 3: DREAM THE DREAM

Let's play a game. Close your eyes and imagine you just found Aladdin's Lamp on the side of the road and out pops the genie, only instead of just three wishes, he offers you unlimited wishes. What would you wish for? What would you want your life to be if you knew it was impossible to fail?

Take all the present circumstances out of the equation for the moment (people, jobs, money, time, etc.—don't worry, you can always add them back in later if you want to)—allow yourself the luxury of dreaming and using your imagination. We know this can be hard at first—we're so conditioned to not use our imagination—to be realistic, to be logical. To hell with logic for now—dream and imagine. What would you really want if you knew you couldn't fail (not what you think you can get, but what you really want with all your heart)? Answer all of the following questions in as much vivid detail as possible (don't be afraid, go grab some additional sheets of paper and let your visions flow out of you onto the paper—it's so good).

1.   What does your dream house look like? How is the floor plan laid out? Take yourself on a tour of the house—what are the furnishings like? What's the view from the bedroom window?

_____

_____

_____

_____

_____

_____

2.   What kind of car do you drive? What does it look like? What features does it have?

_____

_____

_____

_____

3.   Describe your wardrobe?

_____

_____

_____

_____

4.   What kind of vacations do you go on? How often do you go? How do you travel? What type of accommodations do you use?

_____

_____

_____

_____

5.   What do you do for fun?

_____

_____

_____

_____

6.   How do you help others?

_____

_____

_____

_____

7.   What is your purpose in life?

_____

_____

_____

_____

8.   Who are you with? How do you spend your days?

_____

_____

_____

_____

9.   Describe your ideal day—what would you do on a free day with absolutely no commitments or responsibilities? If you had a day to spend with your kids that was completely unscheduled, what would you do?

_____

_____

_____

_____

10.   Now that you are living your dream life—which emotions are you feeling right now? What are you wearing? Is there a smell in the air? What do you hear? What is your environment?

_____

_____

_____

_____

ALLY'S ANSWERS

What does your dream house look like? How is the floor plan laid out? Take yourself on a tour of the house—what are the furnishings like? What's the view from the bedroom window?

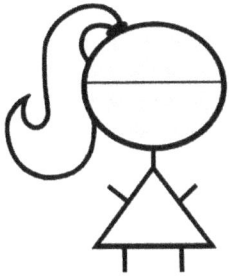

My dream house is on the beach on the Outer Banks of North Carolina. It is a huge expanded Cape Cod style house with weathered grey wood siding. It has six bedrooms, One of which we converted into an office, One is a workout room and one is guest room. The Master bedroom faces the dunes and you can see the ocean beyond. The kitchen is equipped with all of the latest and greatest in culinary technology. The house has a large deck that runs across the entire back of the house, facing the ocean. It is a beautiful, spacious, comfortable and inviting home for my family.

What kind of car do you drive? What does it look like? What features does it have?

I drive a Porsche Cayenne Turbo Tiptronic SUV. It is Amethyst Metallic (kind of a dark plum color). It is loaded with all of the top of the line bells and whistles—GPS, Bose stereo system, etc. It is an AWESOME vehicle!!

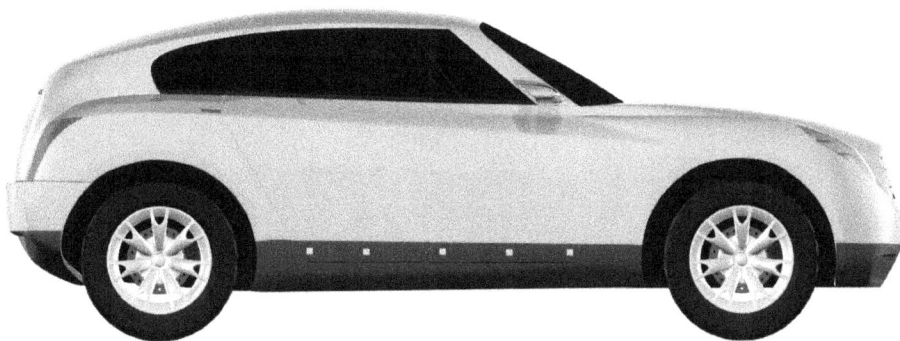

With Hope You Have Options

*"There is no medicine like hope, no incentive so great,
and no tonic so powerful as expectation of something better tomorrow."*
~ Orison Swett Marden

One of the first things you must remember as you go through the stages of getting through your problem is that you are not alone. Others have had and/or are going through the same ordeals as you.

NURTURE OR NATURE?

Did you ever notice how you do certain things just like certain relatives? Of course there's a genetic component, but there is also an environmental component at work. When we were really little, we were quite literally programmed by our parents and the people who were around us most. And it's those programs that cause us to act and feel the way we do all our lives. Think about it, when you were a little kid and you were uncomfortable what did your parents do? They gave you a pacifier or a cookie or whatever it took to make you feel better. So, as little kids we formed the habit of looking to something external to make us feel better and as we grew up, we just upgraded the pacifier. So many women out there are unhappy or dissatisfied or uncomfortable with their lives and are turning to food or alcohol or antidepressants to feel better. The beautiful part is that if that is you, then it's not your fault and the programming can be changed!

Another thing we learned is that within each of us is a mechanism—very much like the autopilot on an airplane—that wants to keep us right where we are. It results in quite the paradox when we find ourselves at a point where we want to change our lives, but that mechanism is doing everything it possibly can to keep us stuck right where we are! Again, this can be traced right back to childhood.

As a baby, you were a born goal achiever! Think about learning to walk—you got up, you fell down, you got bumped and bruised along the way and it didn't matter how many times Mom or Dad gasped and told you, "Be careful! You'll hurt yourself!" You were compelled to walk. Several years later, when you learned to ride a bicycle or to roller skate, your parents were gasping behind you telling you to "be careful so you don't break your neck"! You still learned how to do it, but you started becoming more cautious—worrying that you might indeed fall and break your neck. As you grew even older, you became even more safety conscious. In most every area of your life you were urged to play it safe, weigh the pros and cons, don't take too big a risk. Yet in reality, you are capable of amazing things—is it any wonder you get to middle age and are discontent with the life you've built on that cushion of caution.

Think about it, the life you are living, the feelings you are feeling, the actions you take—they are all the result of the "programs" you received as a small child. It's not that your parents wanted to limit you—they just didn't know any better. But your self–image is a complete result of what was instilled in you by those people around you before you had any clue what was happening. Now it's time to take control and create the self-image you want.

Here's another issue: we are conditioned to treat symptoms rather than find out the cause. You know, a headache is a sign that something is wrong inside your body, it's not a symptom of an aspirin deficiency. Being lonely and miserable is not the symptom of an antidepressant deficiency and being stressed out at the end of the day is not a symptom of a wine or scotch deficiency!

Again, everything we do and every result we are getting is being driven by our belief system and the programming we received as a child. That self-image, that belief system, is nothing more than a huge collection of habits—paradigms—the programming. Remember, it's happening in the background and without your permission like that nasty computer virus. But it really is possible and actually quite simple to re-program your "hard drive" with clean, virus-free programs—and YOU get to choose them this time around!

Let's spend a few minutes digging down into this thing called "the mind" and fleshing out what paradigms are. Pay attention! This is the heart of the program—if you can understand the role of your mind and your paradigms in the results you are getting—you will be able to change anything and everything you choose!

THE MIND

When most individuals talk about the mind and brain, they use the terms interchangeably. In actuality, they are very different and distinct. We like to describe the brain as the radio and the mind as the music. The music is transmitted through the radio; it doesn't originate from it. Much in the same manner the brain is the biological organ inside the skull and our thoughts don't originate from it. For most people, say "mind" and they think "brain." The brain is on the physical plane; the mind is an activity found in every cell of our being; it is on the spiritual plane and it can be divided into two separate sections: the Conscious Mind and the Subconscious Mind.

When we are working with our clients, we start by making the distinction between the mind and the brain, but we have to add a visual image of what the mind "looks" like. See, when you and I think, we literally think in pictures. And the clearer the picture we have of something, the more order and the less fear, doubt, and confusion we will experience.

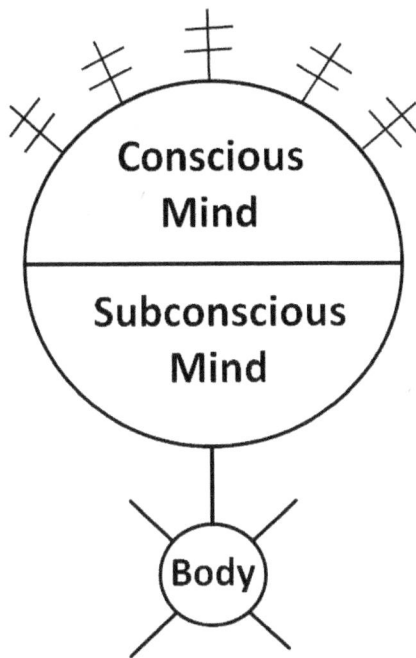

THE STICK PERSON

In 1934, Dr. Thurman Fleet, chiropractor and founder of the Concept Therapy Institute, was working with his patients to literally "think" themselves well. He kept running up against a roadblock when discussing with them the mind's role in healing the body. They had no visual frame of reference for the concept of "mind." Dr. Fleet decided that since our thoughts are visual, we need a picture of our mind. As a result of his decision, a very simple yet profound tool known as the "Stick Person" emerged. Dr. Fleet's drawing brings order and understanding to our mind and is a helpful means of explaining how our thoughts affect how we see ourselves, and ultimately determine our results. This image is the best explanation of how each level of your mind works together with your body to give you your results in life. So now, let's take a closer look at the Stick Person.

We start with a version of the stick figure person that every one of us drew a million times in kindergarten, only in this version the head is purposely drawn disproportionately larger than the body. This is because the mind is dominant over our lives, not the body; the body is merely an instrument of the mind. Then we add a horizontal line bisecting the head into two halves. The top half of the head is the Conscious Mind, or our thinking mind and the lower half is the Subconscious Mind, or our emotional mind. We take in information from the outside world through our five senses (sight, hearing, taste, touch and smell), which are hardwired into our conscious mind like little psychic antennae. The input from our physical senses evokes thoughts (in our conscious mind) which cause us to experience feelings (in our subconscious mind), which drive the body into action, which in turn leads us to the results we are getting in our lives. What we want you to start understanding is that our results are ultimately driven by our thoughts, so if you can change your thoughts to produce different feelings to drive your body into different actions, you cannot fail to achieve different results!

PARADIGMS

Paradigms are a collection of habits or beliefs. Most of our paradigms are formed early in childhood, based on the way we were raised. Paradigms can be good (the paradigm that you pay yourself first so you can amass a large amount of savings) or bad (the paradigm that money is the root of all evil). Paradigms are stored in our subconscious mind. They were installed when we were very young—before our conscious minds ever formed. The "bad" ones are the "computer viruses" that are holding us back. As babies whatever was going on around us—our parents' conversations, the TV news, the nanny's telephone calls—everything we were exposed to was just dumped into our wide open subconscious minds. Over time, just like we learned our name by the repetition of others using it, our paradigms were formed as conversations and themes were repeated in our surrounding environments. So you can see the problem right? Our paradigms—the very things that are holding us back from living the life we were destined for—are other people's habits! We had nothing to do with what got dumped into our subconscious minds as babies. And you know what—that just plain stinks!

So we grow up with all these hang ups and have no clue where they came from. Well, you can thank dear old Mom and Dad (and Grandma and Grandpa and dear Aunt Sally and Uncle Matt and whoever else you spent a lot of time around as a baby). Now don't go getting mad at us—we're not dissing your parents—they had no clue what they were doing. They, no doubt, thought they were doing the very best for you, but the fact remains that your paradigms have very little to do with you. On the flip side, we're also not giving you license to play the victim either! You have been gifted with an intellect and with free will and you had the power to change your life all along, you just didn't know it! There is hope; you can reprogram your paradigms—you can wipe the hard drive of all the unhealthy programs that aren't serving you well and replace them with new ones that will give you everything you want in life!

If you want to know what your paradigms are you have only to look at the present results in your life. Remember that your thoughts in your conscious mind lead to feelings in your subconscious mind (where the paradigms live); those feelings drive the body into action and it's the action the produces the results. So you see you can trace your results directly back to the feelings that are evoked by the paradigms in your subconscious mind. If you can reprogram the paradigms that are no longer serving you then, by law, you can't help but change your results!

So, you may be asking, "What's the key to re-programming your paradigms?" (We're so glad you asked!) Repetition is the key! Any subconscious habit or set of habits can be removed and replaced through repetition.

A 30-day NASA experiment demonstrated the importance of repetition. Astronauts went through experimental training to help them overcome the disorientation from space travel. This training required them to wear glasses that made them see everything upside down for 30 days. The glasses were to be worn 24/7. After thirty days, an amazing thing happened; the mind reprogrammed itself and flipped everything right side up again. But, if at any time one of the astronauts removed the glasses, the mind returned to its original way of thinking. Those who removed them during the experiment had to start all over again and had to wear them for a consecutive 30 days to experience this phenomenon.

The NASA experiment teaches us the absolute necessity of repetition to change our thoughts. We can't be gung-ho one day and sit on the couch the next. If you want to change your thoughts, you have to reprogram your subconscious for a consistent 30 days, even on weekends and holidays. It takes 30 days to form a new habit —that's 30 consecutive, no cheating days in a row. One of our favorite sayings is "do the things you have to do until you want to, then once you want to you will never have to again."

EXERCISE 4: PARADIGM PARALYSIS

The nasty thing about paradigms—the bad ones, at any rate—is that you had very little or nothing to do with establishing them. Your paradigms are generations old—they are your parents' and your grandparents' and your great grandparents' even. It is a shame that something as potentially enabling or crippling as your belief system and your self-image were not of your own choosing—that is, until now!

Think about some of your beliefs that are holding you back. Identify three paradigms that you know aren't serving you in your life.

1. _____

_____

_____

2. _____

_____

_____

3. _____

_____

_____

ALLY'S ANSWERS

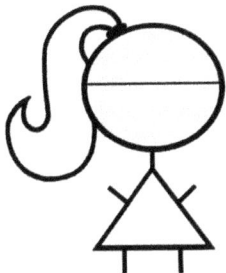

Money is the root of all evil. How many times did I hear my Grandpa say that when I was growing up?

You have to have a college education to get anywhere in life. Mom and Dad both said this all the time. I didn't even know people didn't go to college until I was about 12 years old.

You have to work long, hard hours to get ahead in life. Again, my Dad's motto—never work SMARTER, just work HARDER.

SIX INTELLECTUAL FACULTIES

Ask any first-grader to list their five senses and they can do it without skipping a beat. Our physical senses are incredibly important in our lives, but there is another group of faculties, which are infinitely more important, that most people don't have a clue about. We dare say if you got a group of 100 of the most brilliant PhDs in a room and asked them to list their six intellectual faculties that 98 of them would be unable to do so. Our intellectual faculties are very much like mental muscles and, just like physical muscles, they can be developed and made stronger through regular exercise. And when used properly, will enhance our thoughts and produce really whatever it is that we want in our lives.

Unfortunately, again, this is not stuff that is taught in the average school system—although it certainly should be! Your six Intellectual Faculties are:

1. Will

2. Imagination

3. Perception

4. Reason

5. Intuition

6. Memory

These faculties are always at work, but more often than not, we unconsciously use them against ourselves because of our conditioning. Your ability to create the life of your dreams starts with your decisions. The ability to make sound decisions is directly related to the development, integration, and strength of these Intellectual Faculties, which, when exercised, expand infinitely. Let's take a look at these Intellectual Faculties individually.

WILL

The Will is the intellectual faculty that gives your mind real power. The Will is the ability to focus intently. It's the ability to hold your goal or your vision or your purpose on the screen of your conscious mind over time so that the vision can begin to seep down into your subconscious. It is your ability to concentrate, your ability to stay focused on one thing to the exclusion of all outside distractions. The Will is to the mind what a magnifying glass is to the sun. If you lie in the sun for a couple of hours, you'll get a nice golden brown tan from the sun's rays; however, if you harness those same rays through a magnifying glass, you'll blister your skin in about six seconds. It's the same energy; it's just focused. And that's what you have the ability to do with your Will, by holding your dreams on the screen of your mind with focused intensity.

IMAGINATION

Imagination is your ability to mentally create. Napoleon Hill wrote in *Think and Grow Rich* that the imagination is the most marvellous, miraculous, inconceivable force the world has ever known. You have a brilliant imagination — right now— so start using it! Understand that everything counts, everything is fair game, there is nothing that you can imagine that can't come to fruition somehow. Build pictures in your mind of how you want to live — totally ignore what you may consider to be your present constraints or obstacles — let your imagination take flight and concentrate on building the image of exactly how you want to live. Your imagination is a powerful force that can either work for or against you. You can either imagine how you can accomplish a goal or how you can't.

PERCEPTION

Perception is the lens through which you see the world. Everyone approaches everything they come across in their life — every problem, opportunity, idea, and person — from their own point-of-view and through their own perception. And just because my perception of a situation is different than yours doesn't mean that I'm right and you're wrong (or vice versa). Perception is your ability to see the world. For every good there is a bad, for every up there is a down, and for every hot there is a cold. With this knowledge, you can use your perception to view something as an obstacle or you can look at it as a chance for growth and look for the possibilities. Never underestimate the role of perception in your daily life. It has the power to alter your attitude and course of direction almost without your notice. Visualize and perceive what you want your perfect life to be and soon your perception will help you manifest it into reality. When you change the way you look at life, your life changes.

REASON

Reason is the God-like part of you where you can think and choose. It is actually your free will and what separates you from the animals. This is the higher side of your own nature. We are the only species that have the ability to reason. Reason is your ability to think and all great leaders throughout history, who agreed on nothing else, have agreed that we become what we think about. Your reasoning factor gives you the conscious ability to take a power that flows into your consciousness and literally create a thought. As one thought builds upon another, ideas are formed. But also be warned, when you base your decisions on Reason (and logic) alone, you will quickly reject anything that doesn't match your current understanding or paradigms. This guarantees that you will continue to act on ideas that keep that paradigm in place, and are likely to reject an idea that would move your life or dreams forward. Reason gives birth to thoughts and ideas, but you also need to look to your other intellectual faculties to process and evaluate those ideas — ideas that can and will change your life!

INTUITION

Your intuitive factor can be the greatest tool you have, but you have to decide to develop it! Intuition is the mental faculty that allows you to literally tune into the vibrations of the universe. You transmit vibrations all day long—thought is energy and when you think you transmit energy—thoughts are omnipresent. Intuition seems magical, so much so that some people call it a sixth sense or a coincidence or a hunch. Intuition is an incredibly powerful tool if you take the time to develop it. Intuition is also that "little voice" that speaks to you, trying to guide you toward your true purpose. If you are to truly be successful then you must develop this faculty.

MEMORY

Did you know that you have a perfect memory? Everyone does! There are just a lot of people walking around who say they have a bad memory. The problem is you are likely using your memory incorrectly. Women tend to be emotional "ruminators." Rather than considering what might happen in the future, we tend to dwell on what has happened in the past (which, of course, we can't change), actually perpetuating more of the same into the future! What you need to do is use your memory to focus on the good in your life. You can remember all the successes you've had in your life. You can remember all the great things that you have accomplished and all the obstacles that you've overcome. It is imperative that you stop allowing those negative memories to control the way you are thinking, because they will ultimately control what will manifest in your life.

Now, imagine the possibilities if you were to develop all six of these intellectual faculties and put them to use for you instead of against you. You have infinite potential and you really do have the ability to create your life. And that's exciting!

EXERCISE 5: 20/20 HINDSIGHT

Think back over your life—give one example of an instance where you have used each of your intellectual faculties in a way that really impacted the results you were getting in your life. To illustrate the power of them, in each instance think about whether you used the faculty for or against yourself. Really think about it. For example, have you ever let your perception cloud your decision-making? Have you ever pre-judged a person based on what they look like or how they speak? Have you ever heard that little voice of intuition and listened to it? Have you ever pulled a statistic or something you learned years ago out of the air just when you needed it, even though you thought you had forgotten it long ago? How has your will served you in the past?

Will:

_____

_____

Imagination:

_____

_____

Perception:

_____

_____

Reason:

_____

_____

Intuition:

_____

_____

Memory:

_____

_____

THE TERROR BARRIER—WHEN CHANGE SCARES THE HELL OUT OF YOU!

Okay, so you've read the book to this point and completed the exercises and agree that the concepts make sense. You decide to make some changes in your life. Let's say you've decided to go back to school—maybe it's been your dream since childhood to be a nurse and you've decided to apply to a nursing program at a local university. As long as you just noodle with the idea in your conscious mind everything is cool. But as you start to really focus on this big new idea and think about it more and more and attach emotion to it, the new idea starts to seep down into your subconscious mind. It's at this point that all hell can break loose! You see, your paradigms, your conditioning, your self-image live in your subconscious mind—let's call the paradigm "Mr. X."

In your normal state, your conscious mind thought "X" type thoughts, which produced "X" type feelings (which resonated strongly with Mr. X—your "X" type conditioning), which drove your body into predictable "X" type actions, producing predictable "X" type results. Now, you've suddenly dreamed up this brilliant, shiny, new "Y" type thought (going back to school) that just won't go away. You've become emotionally involved with the idea and your conscious mind starts impressing this new idea on your subconscious mind where Mr. X lives—that's where the trouble starts. Mr. X doesn't like to share and has no intention of having a roommate, so he starts to play dirty. He starts whispering in your ear that this new idea just isn't for you. How on earth are you going to pay college tuition? Where are you going to find the time to study? How could you be so selfish as to neglect your children for such a foolhardy endeavour? Besides, you probably couldn't pass the tests any way—you're really not that bright you know. All of Mr. X's harping starts to generate thoughts of doubt and worry, which generate feelings of fear, which drive your body into a state of even more anxiety than you're already feeling. At that point, without the awareness of what's happening, you will generally retreat right back to the safety of your "X" conditioning and dismiss the "Y" idea as mere folly—and dismiss this program as making your anxiety even worse than when it started—thanks a lot Deb and Angie! Mr. X will go to extreme lengths to maintain control and kick out Mr. Y. He wants nothing more than for you to stay stuck right where you are! Don't let Mr. X win. If you can become more and more emotionally involved with that "Y" idea and how it is going to improve your life and keep thinking and emotionalizing those "Y" thoughts, over time Mr. Y will get stronger and Mr. X will get weaker. As time passes, Mr. Y has a better and better chance of winning what was once an impossible battle. When Mr. Y wins, that is when your paradigm is changed and you now think "Y" thoughts and feel "Y" feelings and act in a "Y" way and consequently get "Y" results—you've broken through the Terror Barrier!

EXERCISE 6: IDENTIFY THE DREAM STOPPERS

Identify ten major circumstances or obstacles in your life that you feel are keeping you stuck. Do not give any energy at all to the insurmountable nature of the obstacles. Do not allow guilt to come into play. Be honest; what do you think is holding you back? Write it down even if you think "you shouldn't feel that way". For instance, it's okay to list your children or your spouse. You are dealing with perceptions and you will not be able to change them until you identify them.

1._____

2._____

3._____

4._____

5._____

6._____

7._____

8._____

9._____

10._____

ALLY'S ANSWERS

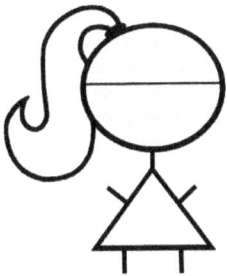

I can't quit my job—we need my income

My kids have so many activities I have no time for myself

I have no time to work out

We can't afford a gym membership so I can exercise to get healthy

I am so stressed out all the time

My husband must think I'm gross, he hasn't come near me in ages

I wish I could go back to law school, but there's no money and no time as it is

My husband doesn't help around the house at all

I am exhausted all the time—I need to eat better

I can't sleep—I wake up in the middle of the night and stress over everything that is wrong in my life.

EXERCISE 7: STOP THE DREAM STOPPERS WITH AFFIRMATIONS

An affirmation is a short, concise statement that, when repeated over and over again, can be used to change your thinking on a subject from negative to positive. Using positive affirmation statements forces you to keep focused on your goals and reminds you to think consciously about your words and thoughts and to modify them to reflect a positive attitude.

There are a couple of important components of an affirmation. First, you want to be in the right headspace—a state of happiness and gratitude. Gratitude opens you to spirit and spirit flowing through you is what will make for lasting change. Second, you must word your affirmation in the present tense as if it were already fact. Remember, the subconscious mind has no ability to distinguish between reality and fantasy, so if you impress the idea that your affirmation is already a fact, it has no choice but to accept the affirmation as actual fact and move the body into action to manifest that result.

You can use affirmations to help change habits/beliefs/paradigms that are not serving you. For instance, if you—like Angie—are finding yourself at the bottom of a bottle of wine more nights than not, your affirmation might go something like this: "I am so happy and grateful now that I have a cup of herbal tea to relax me before bed and save the wine for special occasions and celebrations."

Let's take another example—perhaps one that is even more difficult for you. Let's say that you have identified that you are spending so much time shuttling your children to all of their various after-school activities that you can't get a proper dinner on the table and get home late and are frazzled every single night. Although it was hard to even write the words, you identified the time your children take away from your schedule as one of your ten things that are holding you back. Create an affirmation (and yes, we, your faithful authors use this one every single day) something like: "I'm so happy and grateful now that I always have time and energy for the things and people who are important to me." It may seem silly, but it works!! Try it for 30 days and see for yourself!

Now, using the steps in the paragraph above, take the ten circumstances or obstacles that you identified earlier and create an affirmation that turns the negative into a positive.

1. _____
   _____

2. _____
   _____

3. _____
   _____

4. _____
   _____

5. _____
   _____

6. _____
   _____

7. _____
   _____

8. _____
   _____

9. _____

_____

10. _____

_____

ALLY'S ANSWERS

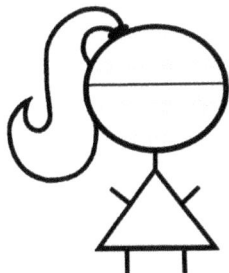

I am so happy and grateful now that I am able to work as much or as little as I choose now that we have more than enough money for me to do as I please.

I am so happy and grateful now that I have time for all the things that are important to me.

I am so happy and grateful now that I have carved out a non-negotiable block of time in my day for exercise four days each week.

I'm so happy and grateful now that I can easily afford a membership at the local health club and that exercising there four days per week is making me stronger and healthier than I have been in decades!

I am so happy and grateful now that my mind is calm and serene. Creative power flows to and through me easily.

I am so happy and grateful now that my husband and I have a wonderful physical connection—just like newlyweds!

I am so happy and grateful now that I've been accepted into law school with a full scholarship.

I am so happy and grateful now that my husband and I share equally in the household duties.

I am so happy and grateful now that my diet is wonderfully varied and healthy and that I have more energy than ever before!

I am so happy and grateful now that I sleep eight hours per night and go to sleep easily and awake refreshed in the morning, ready to tackle the day.

Decision and Action

There is one single action you can take which will propel your life forward like nothing else can. It has the potential to alter the course of your destiny in ways you never thought imaginable—it's called decision. No matter how you look at it, the truth is that decisions are responsible for the results we get in our lives. Even when you don't make a decision, you have in reality made a decision to not make a decision. We have been taught from a very early age to look at the pros and cons, analyze the situation carefully, look at all of the "what ifs." But what you need to understand is that your logic is driven by your paradigms, by your experience, and by your past. You must learn to acknowledge logic and take what is relevant, but not let it control you. To grow and live and prosper you must be willing to be illogical. Those who have become very proficient at making decisions, without being influenced by the opinions of others, are the same people who appear to "have it all" to the outside world. Our entire lives are dominated by the power of sound decisions. When you make a decision, commit to it and don't give up. We need to make decisions quickly and efficiently; you must learn to decide right here, right now with what you've got. Decision-making is a crucial part of all of our lives.

So, now for the good part, the "how." Just how do you make effective decisions? Our favorite tools are:

1. The Four Questions

2. The 3–3–3 Approach

Let's go through each of these techniques:

THE FOUR QUESTIONS

Use the "Four Questions" tool any time you are struggling with a decision. Recall for a moment our discussion of the Terror Barrier. Remember Mr. X and how he can play really nasty games in your subconscious mind as you entertain these new big ideas? Again, one of the questions we get all the time goes something like this:

"When that little voice inside my head starts talking to me about my new idea, how do I know if I am experiencing a burst of inspiration through intuition or if Mr. X is just messing with my mind?" To answer this question, you have to ask yourself four more questions:

1. Do I want to be, do or have this?

2. Will being, doing or having this move me in the direction of my goal?

3. Is being, doing or having this in harmony with God's laws or the laws of the Universe?

4. Will being, doing or having this violate the rights of others?

If you answer "Yes" to questions one, two, and three, and "No" to question four, then you can feel confident that you should decide to keep moving forward. Don't worry about "how" you are going to move forward, no matter how impossible it may seem. That's where the "3-3-3" approach comes in.

ALLY'S ANSWERS

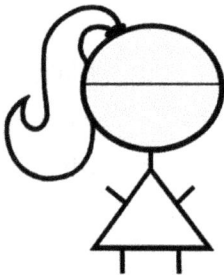

Ally has a nagging desire to go back to law school. She has been a paralegal at a large law firm for 15 years and knows that she would make an outstanding attorney, but dismissed the idea for a myriad of reasons. The idea won't go away— especially now that her children are teenagers and don't need as much of her time as they did when they were little. She continues to struggle with the decision to even make the first move on her idea.

1. Do I want to be, do or have this? Yes

2. Will being, doing or having this move me in the direction of my goal? Yes

3. Is being, doing or having this in harmony with God's laws or the laws of the Universe? Yes

4. Will being, doing or having this violate the rights of others? No.

THE "3-3-3" APPROACH

In his book *You Were Born Rich*, Bob Proctor relates a story about Bob Templeton, a man who was an executive in a telecommunications company that owned radio stations across Canada. He had witnessed the aftermath of a devastating tornado in the town of Barrie, Ontario and he wanted to do something to help the people in the town. He decided that he was going to figure out a way to raise a large sum of money immediately to give to the town of Barrie. The next week he called all of the top executives in the company into a meeting and asked them if they wanted to raise three million dollars, three days hence in only three hours, and give the money to the town. The people in the meeting began spitting out all the reasons why this was an insane idea, but Templeton stopped them saying, "I didn't ask you if we could, or even if we should, I asked you if you would like to." Of course, everyone's charitable nature wanted to help the town, so Templeton took a page of a large flip chart and drew a big "T" on the page. On the left side of the T he wrote "Why We Can't" and on the right side of the T he wrote "How We Can." Then, on the "Why We Can't" side of the chart he drew a big "X" that encompassed the whole column.

Templeton was aware of both the Law of Polarity—for every up there's a down, for every good there's a bad, and for every reason why we can't there is a reason why we can—and the power of perception. So, he told the people in the meeting that there was no room to write down any reasons why they couldn't raise the money in the specified time—regardless of how valid the reasons might be — and if someone brought up a reason why it couldn't be done, the rest of the room was to say "next" until a positive idea came up. By concentrating on how they could achieve their objective, the Telemedia Company indeed raised over $3 million during a three hour trans–Canada radio–thon, which occurred three days after that fateful meeting. The basis of this decision-making and brainstorming tool comes in focusing 100% of your attention on how you CAN accomplish something—even if the method of accomplishing it seems completely outlandish. You are not allowed to spend any energy on why you can't accomplish whatever it is you are pondering. We use this method in our business all the time and it is truly amazing how we have moved from what seemed to be a completely unworkable, blocked situation to a solution (usually in the most improbable way) over and over again. By using this concept you can have whatever you want! Put your focus on how you can and "next" every idea telling you why you can't. It is a difficult exercise in the beginning, but you will find that positive ideas will start racing into your mind! Remember, you don't have to know the whole plan. Just make the decision and the steps will become apparent to you as you go along.

Decision-making will propel you forward toward your dreams. Indecision generally occurs when a person is moving contrary to his or her own core values and beliefs. Indecision is crippling in your personal and professional life. If you haven't already, then make the decision right now that you will apply the principles in this book and that you are finished with living a depressed, anxious, limited life forever! Hold on to that vision and positive ways to improve everything will begin to flow into your mind. You don't have to know all the steps to get you where you want to go—in fact, you absolutely shouldn't.

Take a look at the diagram on the next page. This is an adaptation of a slide we use in just about every coaching group or seminar we present because it is so powerfully illustrative of this point. Imagine that the horizontal lines on the diagram are lines of vibration (and there are an infinite number of lines). Currently you are thinking thoughts that are on the lower levels of vibration (the lower row of "clouds") which are consistent with your current level of awareness. These thoughts are ultimately causing your present results through the Law of Attraction. When you make the committed decision to go after some brand new goal (like going back to school to get your nursing degree), your awareness immediately begins to shift to higher levels of vibration, so your thoughts are also on a higher level and new ideas begin to come into your mind. It is here that the next step will become apparent to you. When you take that step, your awareness shifts higher still and the next step comes to you. This process repeats itself over and over again until your awareness is at a level consistent with your goal—and suddenly you find yourself in a cap and gown, walking across a stage receiving your nursing diploma! So don't get wrapped up in the fact that you can't see how you can possibly turn your vision into reality at this point. There's no way you could— and if you can, then your goal isn't big enough and you'll just be moving sideways.

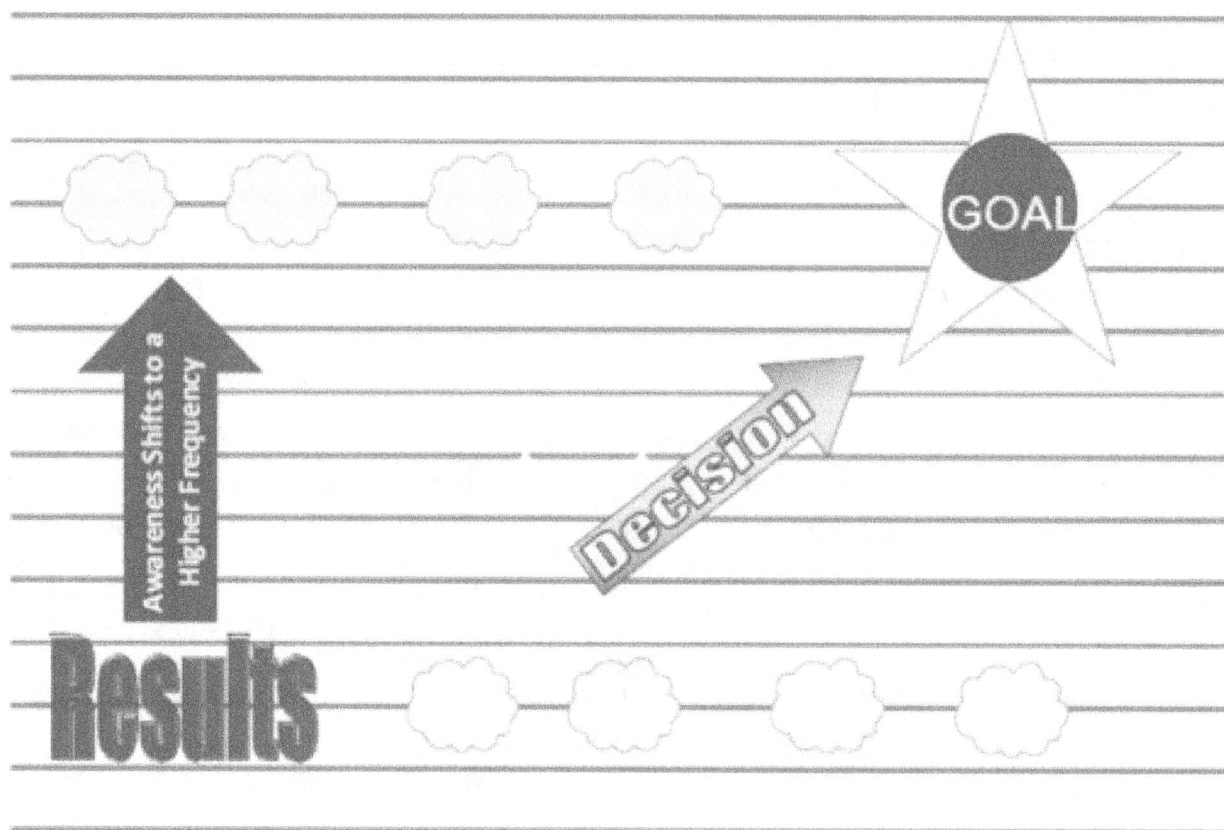

EXERCISE 8: HABITS AND PARADIGMS

Go back to Exercise 3 and look at all the dreams you have for your ideal life. Pick one of these dreams – the bigger and more illogical the better – and use the 3-3-3 concept to brainstorm ways you can move in the direction of bringing it into reality. Give no energy whatsoever to why you can't have what you want, only think in terms of how you CAN. Throw logic and reason out the window – it does not matter how crazy it may sound – one crazy idea may spur several that are not so crazy at all. On the next page, write down whatever comes to mind that could work, no matter how illogical, unlikely or improbable. Then decide from that list what the first step should be and just DO IT! Remember, you have Aladdin's Lamp in your hands – anything is possible, nothing is out of bounds. Get started, move into action!

WHY I CAN'T	HOW I CAN

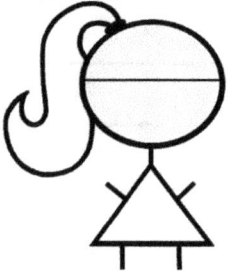

ALLY'S ANSWERS

Ally decided to "3–3–3" her desire to go back to law school

WHY I CAN'T	HOW I CAN
	• Apply to schools I am interested in
	• Complete FAFSA
	• Research grants for women in my situation
	• Talk to manager about part-time or flex-time work (job share)
	• Sell stocks
	• Downsize house
	• Make appointment with financial aid counselor at university to evaluate options
	• Make appointment with bank to see about getting a low interest student loan
	• Research scholarship opportunities for older, female law students
	• Talk to older graduate students to see what they have done

Simple Solutions

Up to this point, the lessons and exercises in this book have been designed to get you thinking (and feeling) in a whole new way—to snap the missing piece of the puzzle into place that shows the reason why people can **know** one thing, but **do** something completely different. The source of the great majority of life's frustrations can be found in that "knowing–doing gap." You may be asking yourself "Where do I go from here?" It's simple—D.R.E.A.M!! Now it's time to take everything from the previous chapters and put it all together into a duplicable simple solution for success.

D = DECIDE

Decide to dream. Decide what you want in life—what you **really** want, not what you think you can get. Commit that your life is too valuable to live in a state of depression and misery! Decide that you will use the tools in this book to take command of your thoughts and feelings and produce the results you **really** want in your life!

R = RECORD

Record the vision. Record it in ways that draw in as many of your physical senses as possible. This will help drive your vision deep into your subconscious mind (which, as you now know, can make no distinction between fantasy and reality).

E = EXPECT

Expect it. Expect that you **will**—beyond a shadow of a doubt—achieve your goal, manifest your vision. Faith and expectancy are integral pieces of the puzzle. Without them, you will be hard pressed to succeed.

A = AFFIRM

Affirm your way through the day. Repeating positive affirmations throughout the day will help you maintain that essential "attitude of gratitude." Remember, what you think about you bring about, so give **zero** energy and thought to what you **don't** want or what you think you're stuck with.

M = MOVE

Move into action! Make your dreams a reality! Remember, thoughts lead to feelings, which move you into action, which produces your results. The D.R.E.A.M. System is designed to move you through this process in a systematic way, thereby creating a new habit: a habit of creating the life of your dreams!

My D.R.E.A.M. System Action Plan

Here's where the proverbial rubber meets the road. The previous exercises were designed to get you thinking about the possibilities in life, rather than your current circumstantial constraints. Now you get to build your personal D.R.E.A.M. system for your own life. If you will follow the instructions to the letter and really put your best effort into it, you can't fail to achieve amazing things! As we've mentioned before, the system is simple, but not necessarily easy. You must commit the time and energy to complete each section as written—you can't pick and choose the parts you want to do or skip sections and expect anything major to happen.

STEP 1: DECIDE

It is absolutely essential that you make the decision to commit to this Action Plan—to take time for the next 90 days to devote to building your dream. You may be in the habit of skipping over details, assuming they are not terribly important (and in many cases they might not be). However, the details of this system are of the utmost importance! We are asking you for a binding commitment to work with this system for the next 90 days; furthermore, we are asking you to sign your name to that commitment. Please don't take this step lightly—when you sign your name, make it mean something—take it as seriously as signing a mortgage deed or a loan document.

My Commitment

I allocate a special, non-negotiable block of time each day to devote to my D.R.E.A.M. System Action Plan. I review and refine my plan daily. I commit to completing the exercises outlined in this action plan for the next 90 days.

_____

Signature   Date

STEP 2: RECORD

Go back to the game we played earlier and refer to your answers from Exercise 3. Once again, close your eyes and imagine you just found Aladdin's Lamp on the side of the road and out pops the genie, only instead of just three wishes, he offers you unlimited wishes. What would you wish for? What would you want your life to be if you knew it was impossible to fail?

Take all the present circumstances out of the equation for the moment (people, jobs, money, time, etc.—don't worry, you can always add them back in late if you want to)—allow yourself the luxury of dreaming and using your imagination. We know this can be hard at first—we're so conditioned to not use our imagination—to be realistic, to be logical. To hell with logic for now—dream and imagine. What would you really want if you knew you couldn't fail (not what you think you can get, but what you really want with all your heart)?

Now that you have that image, write it down—in the present tense (as if your dream were already reality) and in as much sensory detail as you possibly can. Imagine that you have already achieved your goals. Hold a mental "picture" of your dream life as if it were occurring right at this moment. Imagine the scene in as much detail as possible. Engage as many of the five senses as you can in your visualization and then write it down. Note: This step is so very important! You may be tempted to skip it because it's not necessarily easy, but you see, writing causes thinking—it is the start of the creative process. The birth of your new life starts right here, in this step. When you put your vision of what you want down on paper it is the first physical manifestation of that which you desire. When you build the idea in your mind you possess it on the spiritual and the intellectual planes. When you write it down, you begin to manifest it on the physical plane.

_____

_____

_____

_____

_____

_____

_____

_____

_____

_____

_____

Read your vision statement to yourself **twice** a day (preferably first thing in the morning and last thing at night). Relax and let the feelings it evokes wash over you and penetrate deep into your subconscious. As new details of your vision come to mind, re-write your vision statement (do this often).

Kick things up a notch and purchase a digital voice recorder and actually record yourself reading your vision statement (but emotionalize the reading—unleash your inner Meryl Streep) and actually listen to the recording first thing in the morning and last thing at night.

Develop a vision board with pictures of the things you want or images that are consistent with the life you want to create.

Develop a computer slide show that plays as a screen saver on your computer.

STEP 3: EXPECT

Back in the 1960's, Victor Vroom, a Yale University Professor of Management, developed a motivational theory known as Expectancy Theory. Expectancy Theory proposes that a person will decide to behave or act in a certain way because they are motivated to select a specific behavior over other behaviors due to what they expect the result of that selected behavior will be. It's an interesting concept. If you expect something to happen, you will tend to choose to behave in ways that are consistent with the goal. In the context of the D.R.E.A.M. System, if you expect a particular outcome, you will think the thoughts that generate the feelings that propel you into the actions that will produce the result you desire. You have to have unwavering faith and expectancy that your dream will become reality.

My Expectation

It is my unwavering _expectation_ that the vision I have outlined in my D.R.E.A.M. System will indeed manifest in physical reality. I back my expectation with unceasing _faith_ that it will happen.

_____

Signature   Date

STEP 4: AFFIRM

We have already covered the importance of using positive affirmations. Affirmations are a way of feeding your mind thoughts you want to have instead of what is there now that is keeping you stuck or limited. This type of positive "self–talk," phrased in the present tense and expressed in a sincere state of gratitude, drives your dream down deep into your subconscious mind. Once your subconscious latches on to the idea, feelings will be generated to move you into action. The Law of Attraction responds directly to what is going on in your subconscious mind and using positive affirmations is a great way to plant what you want in this fertile soil!

On a separate sheet of paper create a list of positive affirmations that represent your new life and your new attitude. Use Exercise 7 and the Vision you developed in Step 2 of your D.R.E.A.M. System Action Plan as a resource. Then, write the five most powerful ones in the space below. Transcribe them onto an index card and carry them around with you throughout the day. Repeat them to yourself over and over again. Any time you feel yourself slipping into a negative mindset, take out the affirmation card and read it (you only need to monitor how you are feeling—if you feel "bad," you're in a negative mindset). As you do, close your eyes and feel the gratitude for the dreams you are manifesting. Become emotionally involved with what life is like now that your dreams are becoming physical reality.

I am so happy and grateful now that…

_____

_____

_____

I am so happy and grateful now that…

_____

_____

_____

I am so happy and grateful now that…

_____

_____

_____

_____

I am so happy and grateful now that…

_____

_____

_____

I am so happy and grateful now that…

_____

_____

_____

STEP 5: MOVE

Work with this system every day for 90 days. The habits and paradigms that have gotten you where you currently are were formed over years and years. It will take a great deal of repetition of these new ideas in order to supplant them. Each day make at least one decision (refer to Chapter 5) that will move you toward your dream and act on it. Don't force it—force negates everything. Relax and let spirit flow through your calm mind—it always speaks, you just have to listen. Remember, there is no pause button in life—you are either creating or disintegrating. The decisions you make and the actions you take will continually propel you forward—creating your life.

Purchase a journal and make an entry similar to the following every day:

Day 1: I have reviewed each step of the D.R.E.A.M. system, reaffirming my commitments, rewriting my vision, and updating my affirmations.

I have decided _____

and accomplished _____

to move me toward my dream of _____

_____

_____

_____

_____.

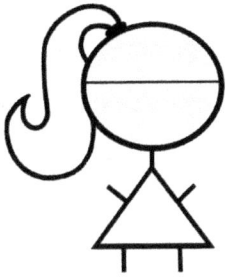

ALLY'S D.R.E.A.M. SYSTEM ACTION PLAN

STEP 1: DECIDE

My Commitment

I allocate a special, non-negotiable block of time each day to devote to my D.R.E.A.M. System Action Plan. I review and refine my plan daily. I commit to completing the exercises outlined in this action plan for the next 90 days.

Allison P. Johnson   12/2/2010

Signature   Date

STEP 2: RECORD

I am so happy and grateful now that...we have income in excess of $1 million/year and are living the life of dreams come true. Jack, Emily, William and I live in a beautiful oceanfront home on the Outer Banks. Our home is warm and inviting to all. As you drive up to the house you pass the three-car garage that houses my fabulous amethyst metallic Porsche Cayenne Turbo SUV, with its buttery tan leather upholstery and every luxury appointment available. The house itself is a two story expanded Cape with weathered grey wood siding and a grey slate roof. Walking into the tiled foyer with its 15' high ceilings, you see a winding staircase that leads to the kids' rooms on the second floor. Beyond, you can see the kitchen with its cherry cabinetry, stainless steel appliances, black granite countertops and huge central island. There is a fully stocked wine cellar and pantry in a room between the refrigerator and the bar area. Past the bar is the living room with its overstuffed, comfortable furniture and 70" LCD television. It's the perfect place to pile in and watch movies together. At the end of the hall is the gym. It has numerous weightlifting and cardio machines and looks out onto the beach. On the other side of the living room is the hallway that leads to the master bedroom, which is spacious and comfortable with its king sized bed, beautiful oak bureaus and armoire and sitting area by the French doors that lead to the private balcony where Jack and I love to watch the sun rise over the ocean each morning and listen to the waves crash on the shore each night. Along the back walls of the living room are *four paneled French doors that lead to the back deck. The kids love to have friends over to lounge around by the pool or head off surfing. Jack and I love to drink coffee or tea in the morning or sip expensive wine in the evening out on the porch and marvel at the magic of our life together.*

Jack is my very best friend, the love of my life, my soul mate. We grow stronger as a couple daily and I am so grateful for every moment we have together. We love to start each day with a vigorous workout and then head for a walk on the beach with the dogs, talking about what new challenges and opportunities await us that day.

I graduated from UNC law school last month and started my own practice immediately. It's been a dream for so long, I can hardly believe it is real! I work out of our home and already have a schedule backlog!! Can you believe it! Jack is able to telecommute from home and only goes into the city twice per month. It has been so amazing for our relationship to be able to work side by side.

Emily will be 17 years old in just a couple of months. She loves living on the beach and she loves her school. She is making exceptional grades in the gifted and talented program, is making new friends easily and it is just a joy to be her Mom. She is excelling in her dance classes and made the varsity gymnastics team at school this year. William just turned 15 and he is all arms, legs and appetite! It seems he grows an inch per week these days! He is learning to surf and just tested for his brown belt in karate. He is an amazing young man.

We are all in excellent health and at elite fitness levels, seemingly aging backwards—wonders to the medical community! I never dreamed I could be so happy and so fulfilled.

STEP 3: EXPECT

My Expectation

It is my unwavering _expectation_ that the vision I have outlined in my D.R.E.A.M. System will indeed manifest in physical reality. I back my expectation with unceasing _faith that it will happen._

Allison P. Johnson   12/2/2010
Signature   Date

STEP 4: AFFIRM

1. *I am so happy and grateful now that I have graduated from law school and established my own successful practice as a family law attorney.*

2. *I am so happy and grateful now that we are living in our dream beach house on the dunes in OBX.*

3. *I am so happy and grateful that Jack's promotion allows him to work from home the majority of the time.*

4. *I am so happy and grateful now that our income is in excess of $1 million/year.*

5. *I am so happy and grateful now that I always have time for the things that are important to me.*

STEP 5: MOVE

Day 1: I have reviewed each step of the D.R.E.A.M. system, reaffirming my commitments, rewriting my vision, and updating my affirmations. I have made an appointment with a financial aid officer at the local university and accomplished a step toward figuring out the financial considerations to move me toward my dream of becoming an attorney specializing in family law.

TAKING RESPONSIBILITY FOR YOUR GROWTH

As you begin to apply the D.R.E.A.M. system, you have to acknowledge that the responsibility for your growth and change falls squarely on your shoulders. In order to stay focused you have to accept responsibility for the choices you make. Responsibility begins with decision. When you refuse to accept responsibility for your life, you will be unable to follow through with any commitments you've made and you end up giving your power over to other people, events, circumstances, or situations. The acceptance of personal responsibility is what separates the winners from the losers. When you fail to take responsibility for your actions, you start to place blame which often leads to a pattern of blaming others and making excuses. Here's the bottom line: Are you happy? If you're not, you need to accept that you're completely responsible for every aspect of your life. Why? Because you chose it freely—no one MADE you do what you're doing or forced you to live the life you're living. If you want to change your life for the better one of the first actions you must take is to assume FULL responsibility for your behavior and thoughts. The more responsibility you assume, the more control you will have.

ACCOUNTABILITY – THE MAGIC INGREDIENT

Accountability is defined as being responsible to someone for some action; answerable. We, your authors, have found accountability to each other to be one the greatest contributing factors to our success. Each week we meet to discuss what our priorities are for the upcoming week and then decide who will do what and we are accountable to each other for those action items throughout the week. And do you know what? We rarely miss a target date. But even more than the activity management advantage of being accountable to each other, we are also accountable to each other for our ATTITUDES. We are all too keenly aware that our attitude – the composite of our thoughts, feelings and actions – will determine our success or failure. Are we perfect? Certainly NOT!! There are plenty of days when one of us wakes up on the wrong side of the bed and nothing is right with the world. But it is at those times that we can look to each other and rise above our current funk. That is the beauty of being surrounded by like-minded people who "get it" and won't let you wallow in your own misery! Let's think about it for a minute, looking back at everything we've covered in this guide… If you wake up one morning smacking up against the terror barrier or are just feeling emotionally down and you can't pull yourself out of your mood, what level are you vibrating on? What are you attracting into your life? That's how you have to think from here on out – how am I feeling and what are those feelings pulling into my life? And if you don't like the answer you have the power to CHANGE your thoughts and feelings IMMEDIATELY!!!

Having an accountability partner can provide that lifeline that you need on those days when you just don't feel like doing it anymore, or damn it, you just want to have a pity party for a minute! Find someone in your life – maybe your spouse, or a good friend, or your Mom or your sister – someone who wants to help you achieve your goal – someone who is like-minded!! Have them read the book and use this system with you over the next 90 days and be your accountability partner. Then when the going gets tough – and it will – you have someone to turn to who will help you see beyond your present mood or give you a kick in the butt when Mr. X causes your resolve to wane. A caveat: The person you choose for your accountability partner should be "like-minded." Make sure they are students of this material as well. There is nothing more difficult than striving to make changes in your life and having your efforts countered (even if subconsciously) by a person who you are looking to help you move forward. Remember, anyone who knows you right now is very comfortable with who you are right now. Regardless of how miserable you may be and how desperately you may want to change and how much they may love you, they are comfortable with who you are today. Despite their conscious intent, their subconscious conditioning will also do anything it can to keep you stuck right where you are. Your accountability partner must be a like-minded student of this material – someone who "gets it!"

Remember, you only get ONE life, make it a life you LOVE, a life that is truly worth dying for!!

What's Next?

So, you've done your self-assessments. You've looked in the mirror. You've allowed yourself to dream again. You learned what Terror Barriers are really all about. You've learned how to Decide, Commit, Record and Expect …

In other words, you're already most of the way to wherever you want to be!

But, we know that sometimes it just doesn't seem that easy or as obvious as we make it sound. We don't want you to get "most of the way" there—we want to see you transform each and every facet of life you wish to transform.

It's why we offer you continued and on-going help and support through our four week online workshop series, *28 Days To YOUR Success Solution*, and other online coaching and consulting packages. These aren't crazy, expensive packages—that's not what we're interested in here. We're interested in:

- Helping you Break Free—getting you past those nasty mental blocks,

- Empowering you to Embrace Change—making congruent decisions with your values, and

- Guiding you to Create a Life you Love—following through on the most efficient and effective action steps to get you there.

We're the added support, the "been there done that" advice and accountability you seek.

Go to our web site at http://www.DebCheslow.com to learn more about what we provide individuals and small groups.

Congratulations, again, for taking this step into the new life you truly deserve.

LEGAL DISCLAIMER

All material provided within *Overcome Dysthmia: Break Free and Create a Life You Love* is for informational and educational purposes only, and is not intended to provide you with medical advice. This workbook is not a substitute for medical care nor is it a substitute for consultation with a healthcare professional. Please discuss all medical questions with your health care provider.

Statements made in *Overcome Dysthmia: Break Free and Create a Life You Love* are the opinions of the authors, based on our research and experience because we have a long running passionate interest in mental health. However, we are not doctors.

The statements made within this workbook have not been evaluated by the Food and Drug Administration. These statements are not intended to diagnose, treat, cure or prevent any disease.

YOU SHOULD ALWAYS SPEAK WITH A HEALTHCARE PROFESSIONAL BEFORE ALTERING ANY PRESCRIBED TREATMENT PROTOCOL.

This workbook was developed by Deb Cheslow Consulting, LLC. The information provided is believed to be accurate at the time it was created and it was based on research and our best judgment. However, like any printed material, information may become outdated over time. Information within this workbook may contain technical inaccuracies or typographical errors, even though we have made our best efforts to avoid any such errors. If there is any doubt as to the accuracy of any claim or information in this workbook, the reader is responsible for verifying same against an alternative source.

All users agree that all use of this workbook is at their own risk. Deb Cheslow Consulting, LLC does not assume any liability for the information contained herein, be it direct, indirect, consequential, special, exemplary, or other damages; including intangible losses, resulting from the use or the inability to use our program.